Ketogenic Instant Pot

Easy Recipes For Healthy Eating To Lose Weight Fast For Smart People

(Ultimate Low Carb Series)

Victoria Westman

<u>**TERMS & CONDITIONS**</u>

No part of this book should be transmitted or reproduced in any form whatsoever, including electronic, print, scanning, photocopying, recording or mechanical without the prior written permission of the author. All the information, ideas and guidelines are for educational purpose only. The writer has tried to ensure the utmost accuracy of the content provided in the book, all the readers are advised to follow instructions at their own risk. The author of this book cannot be held liable for any incidental damage, personal or even commercial caused by misrepresentation of the information given in the book. Readers are encouraged to seek professional help when needed.

TABLE OF CONTENTS

Chapter 1: What Is An Instant Pot?

Basically put, an instant pot is a cooking device that does the work of at least seven different cooking devices put into one.

An instant pot functions as a:

- Slow cooker
- Yoghurt maker
- Pressure cooker
- Warming pot
- Steamer
- Rice cooker
- Saute/browning pan

With the instant pot, you may cook your meals very fast. It cooks meals like dried beans, whole grains, lentils, & stew in about half the time it takes to cook these things with a traditional stove or electric oven.

Do you know that it also functions as a slow cooker so you may prep your meals, place it in your instant pot to cook, set a cooking time & then go about your business to return when your food is done.

This gadget may save you a lot of time & energy, & in case you are wondering if it's healthy, yes it is.

In fact, studies have shown that an instant pot retains 92% more nutrients in vegetables after cooking than traditional stoves & other cooking gadgets because it uses very little water compared to others.

Chapter 2: An Overview Of The Keto Diet

The keto/ ketogenic diet is a high-fat, low-carbohydrate diet that's similar to other low-carbohydrate diets, such as the Atkins diet. This diet focuses on significantly reducing the body's carb intake & substituting it with fat. As a result, the body enters a metabolic state known as ketosis. During this stage, the body becomes extremely efficient at burning fat to make energy & converts the fat in the liver into ketones. In this phase, you won't experience the blood sugar spikes that cause that sluggish feeling a couple of hours after eating a high-carbohydrate meal. It's also in this stage where weight loss happens more easily.

The daily nutritional intake on a ketogenic diet is:

- 5% to 10% from Carbs
- 60% to 80% of calories from Fat
- 20% to 35% from Protein

Chapter 3: Why Follow A Ketogenic Diet?

The most obvious advantage of a keto diet is weight loss. Even though you're not restricting your calories–or even paying attention to them–your body will release the fat you do not need. Weight loss comes with a long list of residual health advantage. You will be at less risk for diabetes, high blood pressure, & heart disease.

In addition to weight loss & a healthier lifestyle, this eating plan is also used to treat illnesses & chronic conditions. It has been effective for people battling epilepsy & children who have suffered from prolonged & dangerous seizures. It also helps to achieve stable blood glucose levels, mostly due to the lack of sugar & carbs in this diet.

Chapter 4: Top 15 Common Myths Of A Ketogenic Diet

1. **For Good Health Carbs are Essential Nutrient:** It's still believed that carbs are necessary to provide glucose to provide energy to the brain & avoid hypoglycemia. But this is not true! Essential nutrients are the ones that your body cannot make on its own, so they've to be consumed on a daily basis through the food sources. There are essential fatty acids & proteins but no such thing as essential carbs.

2. **The Kidneys Suffer Damage from High Protein Consumption during Ketogenic Diets**: This is not true, because, the Ketogenic Diet is not high protein diet; it's a high-fat diet, with adequate protein consumption.

3. **Low-Carbohydrate Diets Lead to Vitamin Deficiencies:** It is believed that low-carbohydrate diets, such as a Ketogenic Diet lead to vitamin deficiencies such as deficiency of vitamin C. But this is not true.

4. **Ketosis is Dangerous:** A Ketogenic Diet leads the body to undergo the method of Ketosis. It's said that Ketosis is a dangerous method, but this is not the case as often Ketosis is confused with Ketoacidosis.

5. **A Ketogenic Diet will Result in Osteoporosis**: It's believed that a high protein & low-carbohydrate diet cause the body to excrete calcium & result in osteoporosis, but a Ketogenic Diet is not a high protein diet! On the contrary, to the myth, high protein intake results in stronger bones.

6. **Low-Carbohydrate Diets Lead to Muscle Wasting**: This is not true. In fact, the low-carbohydrate diets are better at increasing as well as preserving lean muscle mass.

7. **Ketogenic Diets Lead to Degradation in Your Physical Performance:** As athletes take high-carbohydrate diet &, due to this, people believe that low-carbohydrate diet can degrade their physical performance. It's true that, in the start, the body takes the time to adapt; but, slowly, it adapts to burn fat rather than carbohydrate to fuel the body.

8. **A High-Fat Ketogenic Diet Results in Heart Disease***:* This is the biggest myth associated with the Ketogenic Diet. A lot of studies show that on the contrary to what has believed that low-carbohydrate diets improve the heart risk markers over another type of diets.

9. **A Low-Carbohydrate Diet Should Always be Ketogenic***:* No doubt that a Ketogenic Diet is a low-carbohydrate diet, but not all low-carbohydrate diets are Ketogenic. A low-carbohydrate diet may be anything that includes 40 to 100 grams of carbohydrate intake per day & perhaps more, whereas, a Ketogenic Diet is way more specific.

10. **A Ketogenic Diet Lacks Phytonutrients & Antioxidants**: A Ketogenic Diet is a low-carbohydrate diet & not a no-carbohydrate diet! It's possible to fit a good amount of plant food in our diet with a low-carbohydrate intake. A lot of e.g. are seeds, vegetables, nuts, berries, etc. These are all healthy plant foods that you may include in a Ketogenic Diet.

11. **Complex Carbs are crucial to be Included in Your Diet**: It's believed that complex carbohydrates are actually the good carbohydrates & it's crucial to include them in our diet. But this is not so much true.

12. **The Weight Loss from a Ketogenic Diet is Only Water Loss & Not Real Weight Loss***:* For the initial week of a Ketogenic Diet, some of the weight loss is due to water loss. But, after a week or so, the body adapts itself to the Ketones & the

fat loss increases as fats become the major source of fuel.

13. **Ketogenic Diets are Hard to Stick To***:* It's often said that low-carbohydrate diets are difficult to stick to because it tells to avoid certain food items & even groups. But, this is true for all kinds of diets & ultimately people surrender & return to old unhealthy diet again. But, in a Ketogenic Diet, it reduces appetite due to which people eat to the fullest & still lose weight.

14. **As Soon as You Go off the Diet, You Tend to Regain the Lost Weight**: This fact is true to any main diet. If you follow any diet for a short period of time, your body does not adapt itself according to it. But, if you follow the proper diet for an adequate period of time, it becomes a normal behavior. Reducing carbohydrates in the diet should be a permanent change in food habits; & if you return to old eating habits again, it's quite obvious to gain weight.

15. **A Ketogenic Diet is Low in Fiber***:* People who follow a proper Ketogenic Diet eat more fibrous vegetables than following the standard American diet.

Chapter 5: Keto Friendly Food

Below are a lot of examples of what food you should eat when you are on Ketogenic diet:

- Seaweed
- Herbs
- Grass-Fed Butter/ Cream & Ghee
- Coconut Milk and Coconut Milk Yogurt
- Limes and Lemons
- Cheese
- Cottage Cheese & Plain Greek Yogurt
- MCT Oil
- Coconut Milk / Coconut Oil
- Poultry & Meat
- Cocoa Powder & Dark Chocolate
- Olive
- Unsweetened Tea & Coffee
- Olive Oil
- Fish
- Coconut Flour, Butter and Flakes
- Eggs
- Shirataki Noodles
- Low- carbohydrate Vegetables
- Seeds and Nuts
- Avocados
- Berries etc ....

Or Your Shoping List For Keto should be something like this :

- Olive oil
- Macadamia nuts
- Flaxseed (whole or meal)
- Pecans
- Chicken thigh (free range)
- Pumpkin seeds
- Chicken breast (free range)
- Cabbage
- Berries
- Swiss Chard
- Mushrooms
- Full-fat, unsweetened Greek yogurt
- Avocado
- Cucumber
- Soft cheese such as mozzarella or ricotta
- Lettuce
- Coconut oil
- Butter
- Zucchini
- Free range eggs
- Full fat sour cream
- Hard cheese such as cheddar
- Broccoli
- Full-fat cream
- Rhubarb

- Pork chops
- Tomatoes
- Cauliflower
- Eggplant
- Beef mince
- Lamb mince
- Pork mince
- Beef steaks
- Kale

A few advantages here….

Once you have made the change from normal to keto, you will start seeing a whole range of advantage associated with the switch. Your brain thrives on energy derived from ketones, & you won't have to worry about depriving it of anything. The advantage can include the following:

- Boots Energy
- Promotes Clear Skin
- Rapid Weight Loss
- Much Better Sleep
- Better focus

- Reduce Risk of Chronic Diseases
- Keeping Young and Healthy
- And much more ....

Chapter 6: Instant Pot Useful Tips

- **Start with carefully reading the instructions for your device.** Every pressure cooker comes with a manual that you should carefully research, as it contains terms of use, additional useful tips, &, most importantly, information on how use it safely.
- **Store it right.** After finishing your cooking, wash the cooker & put it into storage. Make sure to check the valves & clean those as well.
- **Don't forget to add liquid.** Pressure cooker needs liquid to build up steam pressure inside to actually cook the food. This means you need to make sure to add liquid to the ingredients.
- **Don't overfill the cooker.** All modern pressure cookers have minimum & maximum marks on the inside of the cooking pot. Make sure not to exceed those. When cooking with liquid make sure to avoid filling more than half full, as filling more that may lead to spill.
- **Right heat.** You should make sure to choose the right heat for cooking, as it's 1 of the key elements for successful cooking in the pressure cooker. Check the needed recipe for more details.

- **Right timing.** You should make sure to choose the right timing for cooking, as it's 1 of the key elements for successful cooking in the pressure cooker. Check the needed recipe for more details.
- **Brown the ingredients.** Ingredients in the pressure cooker don't brown, so make sure to actually brown those before you start cooking. If you've a modern electric pressure cooker you may do that in it as well.
- **Slice the ingredients to the right size.** Slice food into even pieces for even cooking. Larger slices will cook slower, smaller slices faster. Check the needed recipe for more details.
- **Release the pressure.** There are generally 2 ways to release steam in your pressure cooker: a) turning a pressure release valve – use oven gloves for this as hot steam will rush out, & c) or open the top lid. However, make sure to carefully open the top lid as not to get burnt.

Chapter 7: The Amazing Keto Swaps

This would not be an ultimate guide if it failed to explain to you how to exactly substitute for your carbohydrate cravings. There are a lot of Keto choices that may be used instead of the unhealthy carbohydrate-loaded ingredients that you can be in the mood of.

Here are the ultimate Keto swaps that will help you maintain the right course:

- All-Purpose Flour ☐ Coconut Flour, Almond Flour
- Rice ☐ Cauliflower Rice (ground ina food processor)
- Baked Goods ☐ You may eat cookies, cakes, bread, & muffins, as long as you substitute the sugar for a sweetener, & the flour for a nut flour. As long as it is low-carbohydrate, you may safely consume it.
- Spaghetti & Pasta ☐ Spiralized Vegetables such as Zoodles (zucchini noodles) or Spaghetti Squash
- Mashed Potatoes ☐ Mashed low-carbohydrate veggies such as Cauliflower
- Bread Crumbs ☐ Ground Nuts
- Lasagna Noodles ☐ Eggplant or Zucchini Slices
- Potato Chips ☐ Zucchini, kale or apple chips

Happy Mashed Cauliflower

Fresh start with something new!!

Ingredients:

- Salt & freshly ground black pepper, to taste
- About 2.5 tablespoons heavy cream
- 1 large head cauliflower (about 3 pounds), cut into large chunks
- About 2.5 tablespoons butter
- 1 cup chicken, beef or vegetable stock

Directions:

1. First of all, please make sure you've all the ingredients available. Pour stock into Instant Pot.
2. Then place cauliflower in steamer basket & set in pot.
3. Season cauliflower to taste with salt & pepper.
4. This step is important. Secure pot lid, close pressure valve & cook properly on steam setting for about 5 to 10 minutes.
5. Now when cooking time ends, let pressure release naturally.
6. Remove cauliflower from steamer basket to a large bowl & add butter and heavy cream.

7. One thing remains to be done. Now mash cauliflower to desired consistency with a fork, potato ricer, or immersion blender.
8. Finally season cauliflower to taste with salt & pepper to serve. Enjoy!

Serves: 4 to 5

Preparation time: 5 to 10 minutes

Cooking time: 15 to 20 minutes

Wow, that's cute!!

Nutrition Information per Serving:

Total Fat: 8g

Sugar: 5g

Saturated Fat: 5g

Fiber: 5g

Protein: 4g

Calories: 128

Carbs: 11g

Reliable Simple Delicious Keto Muffins

Silently, you were waiting for this one. Don't lie... ?

Ingredients:

- 1 cup almond flour
- About 2.5 tablespoon stevia
- 4 tablespoon butter
- 2 tablespoon water
- About 1.5 teaspoon baking soda
- 1 egg
- 1 teaspoon lemon juice
- 6 oz. celery stalk

Directions:

1. First of all, please make sure you've all the ingredients available. Chop the celery stalk roughly and put it in the blender.
2. Then add butter, lemon juice, almond flour, baking soda, egg, water, and stevia.
3. This step is important. Blend the mixture well till you get thick mass.
4. Pour the muffin dough into the muffin forms & put the forms in the instant pot.

5. One thing remains to be done. Close the lid and cook properly the muffins for about 15 to 20 minutes at the pressure mode.
6. Finally when the muffins are cooked – discard them gently from the forms and serve. Enjoy!

Total Time: 25 to 30 Minutes

Servings: 6 to 8

I know, this is amazing!!

Nutrition Information per Serving:

Fat 9.4

Protein 2

Fiber 1

Carbs 1.12

Calories 95

King Sized Simple Artichokes

For those who are not ordinary, try this one.

Ingredients:

- Salt
- Black pepper
- 2 c. water
- About 2.5 tbsps.lemon juice
- 2 minced garlic cloves
- 1/4 c. olive oil
- About 1.5 tsp. dried oregano
- 2 tbsps.balsamic vinegar
- 4 big trimmed artichokes

Directions:

1. First of all, please make sure you've all the ingredients available. Put some water inside your instant pot, add the steamer basket and artichokes, cover & cook properly at high pressure for about 5 to 10 minutes.
2. Now in a bowl, mix lemon juice with vinegar, pepper, oil, salt, garlic & oregano and stir very well.

3.   One thing remains to be done. Then cut artichokes in halves, add them to lemon & vinegar mix, toss well, place them on preheated grill over medium-high heat, cook properly for about 2 to 5 minutes on each side, arrange them on a platter & serve as an appetizer.

4.   Finally enjoy!

Cooking time: 15 to 20 minutes

Servings: 4 to 6

Uber fantastic!!

Nutrition Information per Serving:

Fats: 4g

Protein: 5g

Net carbs: 3g

Calories: 162

Unique One Pot Pressure Cooker Penne Rigate Pasta

Classic, isn't it?

Ingredients:

- 1 small onion sliced
- About 1.5 tablespoon fish sauce, omit if vegetarian/vegan
- 1 small shallot diced (optional)
- 3 cloves garlic minced
- 1 tablespoon Worcestershire sauce, omit if vegetarian/vegan
- 12 white mushrooms sliced
- 1 zucchini squash thickly sliced
- About 2.5 tablespoons light soy sauce
- Dash sherry wine
- Pinch oregano dried
- Pinch basil dried
- Kosher salt to taste
- Black pepper to taste
- 1/2 cup tomato paste 5.5 fl oz can
- Olive oil desired amount
- 1 cup chicken stock or vegetable stock,
- 2 cups Water
- 450 grams penne pasta

Directions:

1. First of all, please make sure you've all the ingredients available. Press Sauté button and click the adjust button to Sauté More function on the Instant Pot. Wait until indicator says "hot".
2. Now if you prefer crunchy zucchini squash, sauté sliced zucchini squash with 1 tablespoon of olive oil and set aside.
3. Flavor Enhancement Step: Add 1 tablespoon of olive oil.
4. Ensure to coat the oil over the whole bottom of the pot. Add minced shallot & sliced onion, then sauté.
5. This step is important. Add a pinch of kosher salt & ground black pepper to season.
6. Then stir occasionally until slightly browned.
7. Add minced garlic & stir for roughly about 30 to 40 seconds until fragrant.
8. Add sliced mushrooms, a pinch of dried oregano, a pinch of dried basil, and sliced zucchini squash (omit zucchini squash if you already sauteed them) & cook properly for another minute. Taste and adjust if necessary.
9. Now pour in a dash of sherry wine & deglaze the bottom of the pot with a wooden spoon.

10.   Mix 1 cup of unsalted homemade chicken stock (or vegetable stock), 2 cups of water, 2 tablespoons of light soy sauce, 1 tablespoon of fish sauce, & 1 tablespoon of Worcestershire sauce in the pot

11.   Now pour penne in the sauce. Place tomato paste on top of the pasta & mix.

12.   Test seasoning and adjust. Ensure all penne are completely submerged in the sauce.

13.   Pressure cook on Manual at High Pressure for about 2 to 5 minutes.

14.   Then turn off the heat and wait 5 to 10 minutes before Quick Releasing the pressure.

15.   Taste pasta, if you find them too hard, close lid & let the leftover heat cook them until desired tenderness.

16.   One thing remains to be done. If you have set aside some crunchy zucchini squash, now is the time to mix them in & serve immediately.

17.   Finally add freshly grated Parmesan cheese to take it up a level. Enjoy!

Prep + Cooking Time: 30 to 35 minutes

Serving: 4 to 6

Different yet fantastic in many ways.

Nutrition Information per Serving:

Total Fat 51 g

Protein 7 g

Cholesterol 0 mg

Total Carbs 42 g

Sodium 10 mg

Calories 509.6

Potassium 0 mg

Energetic Bone Broth

Super awesome plus unique!!

Ingredients:

- 1 small onion, skin on & quartered
- About 2.5 tablespoons apple cider vinegar
- 1" ginger knob
- 3.5-4 quarts water, filtered
- 2 garlic cloves
- About 1.5 chicken carcass, cooked, with most meat drippings removed
- 1 cup celery tops (Chopped)

Directions:

1. First of all, please make sure you've all the ingredients available. Put every solid ingredient into Instant Pot.
2. Then pour water up to the 4 quarts mark.
3. Stir to mix.
4. Close the lid of the instant pot, & set vent to "sealed".
5. This step is important. Press "Manual" button, set the timer for about 55 to 60 minutes & set "Pressure" to high.

6. Now once the timer is up press "Cancel" button & turn the steam release handle to "Venting" position for quick release, until the float valve drops down.
7. Open the lid.
8. NOTE: Please make sure the pressure is fully released before opening the lid, so you simply do not get burnt.
9. Then set broth aside to cool for about 55 to 60 minutes before taking out the solids.
10. Put broth into container & season with sea salt.
11. One thing remains to be done. Refrigerate for up to about 7 to 8 hours or overnight.
12. Finally remove fat from the broth's top.

Cooking Time: 60 to 65 minutes

Servings: 12 to 14

Iconic recipe of my list!!

Nutrition Information per Serving:

Fats (g): 15

Protein (g): 10

Net carbs (g): 2

Calories: 260

Perfect Eggs Sunny Side Up – Keto Style

Be amazed ?

Ingredients:

- 4 eggs
- About 1 tsp rosemary
- 1 1/2 cups cherry tomatoes
- About 2.5 tsp minced garlic
- 1 cup honey-cured bacon

Directions:

1. First of all, please make sure you've all the ingredients available. Cut bacon into 1/2 inch square pieces, & cut cherry tomatoes in half.
2. Now turn the cooker to sauté, set in the inner pot, and then sauté the bacon squares for about 2 to 5 minutes.
3. This step is important. Remove bacon and crack eggs into the pot.
4. Add in the garlic, rosemary, & chopped tomatoes.
5. Then stir in the bacon pieces, cover, seal, and lock.
6. Set cooker to manual and high.
7. One thing remains to be done. Set timer to zero & start.

8. Finally release steam with quick method &
serve hot.

Preparation time: 25 to 30 minutes

Serves: 4 to 5

Wow, just wow!!

Nutrition Information per Serving:

30.6g fat

29.3g protein

4.2g carbohydrates

Ultimate Easy Pork Roast

I know, this is amazing!!

Ingredients:

- About 1.5 tablespoon olive oil
- 4 pounds pork shoulder
- About 1/2 cup keto Jamaican spice mix
- 1/2 cup beef stock

Directions:

1. First of all, please make sure you've all the ingredients available. Then in a bowl, mix pork with oil & spice mix and rub well.
2. Set your instant pot on sauté mode, add pork & brown for a few minutes on each side.
3. One thing remains to be done. Now add stock, cover pot & cook pork shoulder properly on High for about 35 to 40 minutes.
4. Finally slice roast and serve.

Preparation time: 10 to 15 minutes

Cooking time: 45 to 50 minutes

Servings: 12 to 14

Silently, you were waiting for this one. Don't lie… ?

Nutrition Information per Serving:

Fat 6

Protein 16

Fiber 7

Carbs 10

Calories 400

Unique Sausage-Wrapped Eggs

The best combo ever!!

Ingredients:

- 4 Hardboiled Eggs
- About 1.5 tbsp Olive Oil
- 1 cup Water
- 1 pound ground Sausage

Directions:

1. First of all, please make sure you've all the ingredients available. Peel the eggs and divide the sausage into 4 equal pieces.
2. Now flatten each piece of sausage & place an egg on top.
3. Wrap the sausage around the egg completely. Repeat with the remaining eggs and sausage.
4. Heat the oil in the IP on SAUTE & add the eggs.
5. This step is important. Cook properly for about 2 to 5 minutes or until the sausage is slightly browned.
6. Then transfer to a plate.

7.   Pour the water into the Instant Pot & lower the rack.

8.   Arrange the eggs on the rack & close the lid.

9.   Now cook properly for about 5 to 10 minutes on HIGH.

10.   One thing remains to be done. Release the pressure quickly.

11.   Finally serve and enjoy!

Total Time: 20 to 30 MIN

Serves: 4 to 5

Something is new here!!

Nutrition Information per Serving:

Total Fats 50g

Protein 33g

Net Carbs: 2.5g

Calories 615

Best Easy Avocado & Egg Salad

Make me remember the good old days!!

Ingredients:

- 1 large avocado (200 g / 7.1 oz)
- Optional: chives, fresh herbs and extra virgin olive oil for garnish
- About 4.5 cups mixed lettuce such as lamb lettuce, arugula, etc. (120 g / 4.2 oz)
- 1/2 cup soured cream or full-fat yogurt (115 g / 4.1 oz) or 1/4 cup mayonnaise (you can make your own)
- Salt and pepper to taste (i like pink himalayan rock salt)
- 2 cloves garlic, crushed
- 4 large eggs, free-range or organic
- About 2.5 tsp dijon mustard (you can make your own)

Directions:

1. First of all, please make sure you've all the ingredients available. Start by cooking the eggs.
2. Now fill a small saucepan with water up to 3 quarters.
3. Add a good pinch of salt. This will prevent the eggs from cracking.

4. Bring to a boil. Using a spoon or hand, dip each egg in & out of the boiling water - be careful not to get burnt.
5. This step is important. This will prevent the egg from cracking as the temperature change won't be so dramatic.
6. Then to get the eggs hard-boiled, you need round 10 to 15 minutes. This timing works for large eggs.
7. When done, remove from the heat & place in a bowl filled with cold water.
8. I like and always use this egg timer! When the eggs are chilled, peel off the shells.
9. Then make the dressing by mixing the soured cream, crushed garlic and Dijon mustard & season with salt and pepper.
10. Wash and drain the greens in a salad spinner or just by pat drying using a paper towel.
11. Now place the greens in a serving bowl & mix with the dressing.
12. One thing remains to be done. Halve, deseed, peel and slice the avocado & place on top of the greens.

13. Finally add the quartered eggs & season with more salt and pepper to taste. Enjoy!

Prep time: 5 to 10 min

Cooking time: 10 to 15 min

Total time: 15 to 20 min

Serving: 2 to 4

Luxury in its own class!!

Nutrition Information per Serving:

Fiber 7.6 grams

Net Carbs 6.1 grams

Fat 36.3 grams

Protein 17 grams

Total Carbs 13.7 grams

Energetic Sweet Carrots Breakfast

Spice up!!

Ingredients:

- A pinch of cloves, ground
- 1/4 cup pecans (Chopped)
- A pinch of nutmeg, ground
- About 1 teaspoon cinnamon powder
- 1 small zucchini (Grated)
- 2 tablespoons swerve
- About 1.5 carrot, grated
- 1 and 1/2 cups coconut milk

Directions:

1. First of all, please make sure you've all the ingredients available. Now in your instant pot, mix milk with cloves, nutmeg, swerve, zucchini, carrot, cinnamon and pecans, stir, cover & cook properly on High for about 2 to 5 minutes.
2. Finally divide into bowls & serve hot.

Preparation time: 10 to 15 minutes

Cooking time: 5 to 10 minutes

Servings: 4 to 6

What do you think? ?

Nutrition Information per Serving:

Fat 1

Protein 4

Fiber 2

Carbs 3

Calories 100

Ultimate Nutritive Spinach Plate

Stylish.

Ingredients:

- 1 medium yellow onion (Chopped)
- Salt & freshly ground black pepper, to taste
- About 1.5 tablespoon garlic (Minced)
- About 1 teaspoon red pepper flakes, crushed
- 10 cups fresh spinach (Chopped)
- 1 cup tomatoes (Chopped)
- About 1.5 tablespoon fresh lemon juice
- 1/2 cup sugar-free tomato puree
- 11/4 cups homemade vegetable broth
- 2 tablespoons olive oil

Directions:

1. First of all, please make sure you've all the ingredients available. Place the oil in the Instant Pot & select "Sauté".
2. Now add the onion and cook properly for about 2 to 5 minutes.
3. Next, please add garlic & red pepper flakes and then cook for about 2 minutes.

4.   This step is important. Add spinach and cook properly for about 2 to 5 minutes.
5.   Then select "Cancel" and stir in the remaining ingredients.
6.   Next, secure the lid & cook under "Manual" and "High Pressure" for about 5 to 10 minutes.
7.   One thing remains to be done. Select the "Cancel" & carefully do a Quick release.
8.   Finally remove the lid & serve warm.

Makes: 6 to 7servings

Preparation Time: 15 to 20 minutes

Cooking Time: 10 to 15 minutes

Always kept wondering how it was made... One day I sat beside my chef and got it.

Nutritional Information per Serving:

Fat: 5.3g

Protein: 3.4g

Saturated Fat: 0.8g

Sodium: 207mg

Sugar: 3g

Carbohydrates: 7.4g

Calories: 83

Dietary Fiber: 2.3g

Delightful Hearty Bacon & Veggie Soup

Legends are born in…

Ingredients:

- 1 small yellow onion (Chopped)
- 4 dashes hot pepper sauce
- 2 garlic cloves (Minced)
- 1 head cauliflower, chopped roughly
- 6 cooked turkey bacon slices (Chopped)
- About 1.5 green bell pepper, seeded and chopped
- Freshly ground black pepper, to taste
- 1 cup half-and-half
- 4 cups homemade chicken broth
- About 1.5 tablespoon olive oil
- 2 cups cheddar cheese (Shredded)

Directions:

1. First of all, please make sure you've all the ingredients available. Place the oil in the Instant Pot & select "Sauté".
2. Now add the onion and garlic & cook properly for about 2 to 5 minutes.
3. Select the "Cancel" and stir in cauliflower, salt, bell pepper, black pepper and broth.

4. This step is important. Secure the lid and select "Soup" & just use the default time of 15 to 20 minutes.
5. Then select the "Cancel" & carefully do a Quick release.
6. Remove the lid and stir in remaining ingredients.
7. One thing remains to be done. Select "Sauté" & cook properly for about 5 to 10 minutes.
8. Finally serve immediately.

Makes: 6 to 7 servings

Preparation Time: 15 to 20 minutes

Cooking Time: 20 to 25 minutes

Sizzle your taste buds…

Nutritional Information per Serving:

Fat: 32.6g

Protein: 25.8g

Saturated Fat: 15.4g

Sodium: 1444mg

Sugar: 3.3g

Carbohydrates: 8.5g

Calories: 430

Dietary Fiber: 1.7g

Best Instant Pot Delectable Chicken Tikka Masala:

Being lucky is definitely better.

Ingredients:

- 1 diced large onion
- 1/3 cup of chopped cilantro
- About 1.5 teaspoon of coconut oil
- 28 ounces of canned fire roasted diced tomatoes
- 4 cloves of minced garlic
- 3/4 cup of canned coconut milk
- 1 tablespoon of grated ginger
- 2 teaspoons of paprika
- About 2.5 tablespoons of garam masala
- 2 teaspoons of kosher salt
- 2 pounds of skinless and boneless chicken breast

Directions:

1. First of all, please make sure you've all the ingredients available. Turn the sauté

mode in Instant Pot. Add the coconut oil & wait till it melts.

2. Now once the oil is melted, start adding the onions, garam masala, garlic, and ginger, salt, and paprika.

3. You need to cook everything for about 2 to 5 minutes till the onions have softened.

4. This step is important. Turn off the sauté mode.

5. Then add the tomatoes & scrape off everything from the bottom of the pot.

6. Add the chicken and stir it.

7. Combine the masala with the chicken so that all the chicken pieces are well-coated with the ingredients.

8. Now close the lid of the pot & turn on the Poultry mode for about 15 to 20 minutes. Let the chicken cook thoroughly.

9. After the chicken is cooked, let it rest for some time so that the pressure is released naturally.

10. Then open the lid and add the coconut milk. Dip a spoon & taste the masala; adjust the seasonings accordingly.

11. If required, add more curry powder, & salt.

12. Now use the cilantro to garnish the dish.

13. One thing remains to be done. The delicious chicken tikka masala is ready to be served with your favorite roti or nan.

14. Finally it can be served with rice as well; in that case, just increase the amount of gravy in the dish.

Serving size: 3/4-1 cup

Servings per recipe: 4 to 6

Calories: 310 per serving

Calories from fat: 89

Preparation Time: 5 to 10 minutes

Cooking Time: 25 to 30 minutes

Mystery is unveiled!!

Nutrition Information per Serving:

Saturated fat: 11g

Protein: 35g

Sodium: 215mg

Dietary fiber: 4g

Cholesterol: 74mg

Sugar: 5g

Total carbohydrate: 13g

Total fat: 11g

Legendary Spicy Diced Eggs

Classic style…

Ingredients:

- 1/4 tsp smoked paprika
- 11/2 cups water
- About 1 tsp chili powder
- 2 tbsp butter, melt
- 1/4 tsp cayenne pepper
- 1/2 tsp garlic powder
- About 1/2 tsp onion powder
- 1/4 tsp salt
- 1/4 tsp black pepper
- 6 eggs

Directions:

1. First of all, please make sure you've all the ingredients available. Pour the water into your Instant Pot & lower the rack.
2. Then grease a baking dish with cooking spray & crack the eggs into it.
3. Make sure not to break the yolks.
4. This step is important. Cover the dish & place in the Instant Pot.
5. Now close the lid and cook properly on HIGH for about 2 to 5 minutes.

6. Do a quick pressure release & transfer the egg mixture to a cutting board.
7. One thing remains to be done. Dice finely and stir in the spices & butter.
8. Finally serve & enjoy!

Total Time: 15 to 20 MIN

Serves: 4 to 6

Arrive in style with this recipe.

Nutrition Information per Serving:

Fat: 12.4 g

Protein: 8.5 g

Net Carbohydrates: 1.0 g

Calories: 149

Fantastic Cabbage And Carrot Soup

This never goes out of style.

Ingredients:

- 1 chopped small yellow onion
- Ground black pepper
- 12 oz. baby carrots
- About 3.5 chopped celery stalks
- Salt
- 2 tbsps. olive oil
- 4 c. chicken stock
- About 3.5 tsps. minced garlic
- 1 shredded cabbage head
- 1/4 c. chopped cilantro

Directions:

1. First of all, please make sure you've all the ingredients available. Now in your instant pot, mix cabbage with carrots, celery, onion, stock, olive oil and garlic.
2. One thing remains to be done. Then stir the mixture & cover your pot. Next, quickly set the instant pot on High & then cook properly for about 5 to 10 minutes.

3.   Finally add salt, pepper, & cilantro, stir well, ladle into soup bowls & serve.

Cooking time: 10 to 15 minutes

Servings: 4 to 6

Now be a legend!!

Nutrition Information per Serving:

Protein: 10g

Fats: 4g

Calories: 165

Net carbs: 9g

Legendary Orange Chicken Sauce

Prepare yourself for this…

Ingredients:

- 4 chicken breast, cubed
- About 1.5 lemon, sliced into wedges
- 3 garlic cloves (Minced)
- Pinch of ground black pepper
- 1 tsp. dried oregano
- 1 onion, thinly sliced
- 2 tbsp. lime juice, freshly squeezed
- About 1.5 tsp. ground cumin
- 1 bay leaf, crumbled
- 3/4 cup orange juice, freshly squeezed
- 3 tbsp. olive oil (Divided)
- Pinch of salt

Directions:

1. First of all, please make sure you've all the ingredients available. Pour olive oil into the Instant Pot Pressure Cooker.
2. Then press the "saute" button. Cook chicken properly until browned all over. Set aside.
3. Saute onion and garlic for about 2 to 5 minutes or until limp and aromatic. Stir in

dried oregano, bay leaf, lime juice, and orange juice.

4. This step is important. Season with ground cumin, salt, and pepper.
5. Now put back cooked chicken cubes.
6. Lock the lid in place. Press the manual button & cook properly for about 10 to 15 minutes.
7. When the beep sounds, Choose the Quick Pressure Release.
8. Then this will depressurize for about 5 to 10 minutes. Remove the lid.
9. One thing remains to be done. Turn off the crockpot. Adjust seasoning according to your preferred taste.
10. Finally serve with lemon wedges.

Serves: 3 to 4

Recommended serving size: 3/4 cup stew

We all are legends in some ways.

Nutrition Information per Serving:

Protein – 53.94 grams

Sodium – 973 mg

Calories - 410

Carbohydrates – 17.35 grams

Great Pork Chops

Vintage overload…

Ingredients:

- 1 c water
- About 1.5 tbsp coconut oil
- 1 stick butter
- 1 package ranch mix
- 4-6 boneless pork chops

Directions:

1. First of all, please make sure you've all the ingredients available. Set the cooker to sauté & add the coconut oil to the pot.
2. Now brown chops.
3. Add the butter & then sprinkle the ranch packet.
4. Pour the water & place the lid on & lock in place.
5. One thing remains to be done. Then set to manual for about 5 to 10 minutes.
6. Finally let pressure release, then pour over the buttery mix.

Serves: 5 to 7

Prep: 5 to 10 minutes

What do you think?

Nutrition Information per Serving:

Protein: 27g

Net Fat: 16g

Carbohydrates: 4g

Calories: 300

Pinnacle Burrito Casserole

My sister makes it every now & then.

Ingredients:

- 4 large eggs
- 1 c. water with an additional 1 tbsp.
- 1/4 c. chopped yellow onion
- About 1.5 chopped jalapeno
- Keto salsa
- 6 oz. chopped ham
- Salt
- About 1 tsp. taco seasoning
- Black pepper
- 1/4 tsp. chili powder
- 2 lbs. peeled celeriac, cubed

Directions:

1. First of all, please make sure you've all the ingredients available. In a bowl, mix eggs with onion, celeriac, jalapeno, ham, salt, pepper, chili powder & taco seasoning and stir.
2. Now add 1 tablespoon water, stir again & pour everything into a casserole.
3. Next, quickly add the water to your instant pot, then quickly add the trivet, & casserole, cover pot & cook properly on Manual for about 10 to 15 minutes.

4.   One thing remains to be done. Then divide between plates & serve for breakfast with some keto salsa on top.
5.   Finally enjoy!

Servings: 6 to 8

Prep time: 10 to 15 minutes

Cook time: 10 to 15 minutes

Mushroom fries bring back a lot of memories.

Nutrition Information per Serving:

Fat: 4g

Protein: 7g

Carbs: 7g

Calories: 213

Great Broccoli Cheese Soup

Yes, this is famous!!

Ingredients:

- 1 medium onion (Diced)
- 4 cloves garlic, peeled and minced
- About 8.5 ounces Colby cheese (Shredded)
- 4 cups chicken stock
- 1 cup heavy cream
- 4 cups broccoli florets
- 2 tablespoons butter

Directions:

1. First of all, please make sure you've all the ingredients available. In Instant Pot on sauté setting, melt butter and cook onion and garlic until translucent, about 5 to 10 minutes.
2. Then add broccoli and chicken stock to pot & season to taste with salt and pepper.
3. This step is important. Secure pot lid, close pressure valve & cook properly on high setting for about 5 to 10 minutes.
4. Now when cooking time ends, carefully turn venting knob from sealing to venting position for a quick pressure release.
5. One thing remains to be done. Add heavy cream & Colby cheese to soup & stir until cheese is melted.

6. Finally season soup to taste with salt & pepper, serve and enjoy!

Serves: 8 to 9

Preparation time: 15 to 20 minutes

Cooking time: 10 to 15 minutes

Lucky!!

Nutrition Information per Serving:

Total Fat: 22g

Sugar: 2g

Saturated Fat: 15g

Fiber: 4g

Protein: 8g

Calories: 268

Carbs: 5g

Dashing Cheddar Flaxseed Bacon Muffins

Silently waiting…

Ingredients:

- 1/2 cup almond flour
- 2 cups water
- 1/4 cup flaxseed meal
- 2 cored and cubed avocados
- About 1.5 tsp salt
- 1/4 tsp red pepper flakes
- 1/4 tsp garlic powder
- 1 Tbsp lemon juice
- 1 Tbsp chopped green onions
- 1/2 cup shredded cheddar
- 1 cup crispy cooked bacon
- 1 cup coconut milk
- About 1.5 tsp baking powder
- 1 Tbsp baking soda
- 1 tsp black pepper
- 6 eggs
- 3 Tbsp butter

Directions:

1. First of all, please make sure you've all the ingredients available. Spray a dozen silicon muffin holders with food release.

2. Now using a large mixing bowl, combine all ingredients except avocados and stir until smooth.
3. Ladle the batter into each of the muffin holders.
4. This step is important. Arrange muffin holders on top of steaming basket.
5. Garnish each muffin with avocado cubes & cover with foil.
6. Then set cooker to steam & pour in 2 cups of water.
7. Gently place the basket with the muffins in the cooker.
8. One thing remains to be done. Cover, seal, and lock. Cook properly for about 20 to 25 minutes.
9. Finally release steam with quick method & allow muffins to cool on a rack for at least half an hour.

Total Time: 35 to 40 minutes

Serves: 12 to 14

I was waiting for this one

Nutrition Information per Serving:

29.1g fat

14.1g protein

6.4g carbohydrates

Crazy Braised Kale With Green Onions

Cooking level infinite….

Ingredients:

- 2 thinly sliced green onions
- Apple vinegar
- 3 chopped garlic cloves
- Ground pepper
- About 2.5 tbsp. ghee
- Kosher salt
- 1 sliced carrot
- About 1.5 c. water
- 1 lb. chopped fresh kale

Directions:

1. First of all, please make sure you've all the ingredients available. Press the "Sauté" button to heat up the pot & add the ghee.
2. Then toss in the chopped onions, garlic & carrot and sauté until softened.
3. This step is important. Add the kale and water & sprinkle with salt and pepper to taste.

4. Press "Cancel/Keep Warm". Afterwards, press the "Manual" button & the "—" until the display shows "5."
5. Now lock the lid; ensure the valve is pointed towards "Sealing".
6. Allow natural pressure release – let the pressure cooker release pressure naturally without help.
7. One thing remains to be done. Remove the lid, give a good stir, & adjust the seasoning.
8. Finally splash on some apple vinegar & serve.

Cooking time: 15 to 20 minutes

Servings: 4 to 6

Long way to go…

Nutrition Information per Serving:

Fats: 1.12g

Protein: 5.42g

Net Carbs: 7.27g

Calories: 89.14

Ultimate Ginger And Butternut Squash Soup

Yeah, direct from the heaven; yeah?

Ingredients:

- 1 sprig sage
- 1/2 cup pumpkin seeds toasted, for garnish
- 1 large onion roughly chopped
- 1/2 inch piece Ginger peeled and roughly sliced
- Pepper to taste
- About 1/2 teaspoon nutmeg
- Salt to taste
- 4 cups vegetable stock
- Olive oil
- About 4.5 pounds butternut squash peeled, seeded and cubed

Directions:

1. First of all, please make sure you've all the ingredients available. Press Saute to pre-heat the Instant Pot. When "hot" appears on display, add sage, onions, salt & pepper and saute.
2. Now once onions are soft, push onions to the side and add a handful of cubed squash to cover the bottom of the pot.

3. Let the squash brown for about 5 to 10 minutes, stirring infrequently.
4. This step is important. Add the rest of the ginger, squash, nutmeg and the vegetable stock to the pot.
5. Then close & lock the lid of the Instant Pot. Press Manual and then use the [+] or [-] buttons to adjust time to about 10 to 15 minutes pressure cooking time.
6. When time is up, open the pot using Quick Release.
7. One thing remains to be done. Discard the sage stem. With an immersion blender, puree the contents of the Instant Pot.
8. Finally garnish with toasted pumpkin seeds & serve. Enjoy!

Prep + Cooking Time: 20 to 25 minutes

Cooking Time: 15 to 20 minutes

Serving: 6 to 8

What's so typical or different here?

Nutrition Information per Serving:

Total Fat 4.9 g

Protein 5.1 g

Cholesterol 0.0 mg

Sodium 500.2 mg

Total Carbohydrate 32.4 g

Potassium 785.7 mg

Calories 175.0

Funny Spaghetti Squash Chicken Marsala

Well it is a Grandma's recipe!!

Ingredients:

- 2 garlic cloves (Minced)
- Black pepper
- About 1.5 teaspoon coconut oil
- Salt
- 1 cup marsala cooking wine
- Fresh basil
- 1 cup shiitake mushrooms (Sliced)
- 1 cup water
- Large spaghetti squash
- About 3.5 tablespoons xanthan gum
- 1/2 cup organic chicken broth
- 2 pounds chicken thighs or breast, boneless

Directions:

1. First of all, please make sure you've all the ingredients available. Place the steam rack into Instant Pot.
2. Then put spaghetti squash on the steam rack & pour water.

3. Next, please close the lid, and then turn the vent to "Sealed".
4. Quickly press "Manual" button, set the timer for about 25 to 30 minutes and then set "Pressure" to high.
5. Now once the timer is up, press "Cancel" button and allow the pressure to be released naturally, until the float valve drops down.
6. This step is important. Open the lid.
7. NOTE: Please make sure the pressure is fully released before opening the lid, so you do not get burnt.
8. Then take squash out, set aside, pour water out & dry Instant Pot.
9. Put coconut oil into Instant Pot & press "Sauté" button.
10. Put chicken, pepper & salt into Instant Pot and brown the chicken.
11. Now put Marsala wine, mushrooms & garlic over the browned chicken.
12. Next, please close the lid, and then turn the vent to "Sealed".
13. Quickly press "Manual" button, set the timer for about 8 to 10 minutes and set "Pressure" to high.
14. Now once the timer is up press "Cancel" button & turn the steam release

handle to "Venting" position for quick release, until the float valve drops down.

15.   Open the lid.

16.   Then put chicken broth into Instant Pot & stir until evenly mixed.

17.   Take 1/4 cup cooking juice out of Instant Pot & put into a mixing bowl.

18.   Mix 1/4 cup cooking juice with Xanthan Gum until it dissolves.

19.   Now put the Xanthan Gum mixture into Instant Pot.

20.   Slice spaghetti squash into two & get rid of squash seeds.

21.   One thing remains to be done. Peel off squash rind with a fork.

22.   Finally top with mushrooms, Marsala sauce, chicken & garnish with fresh basil.

Cooking Time: 25 to 30 minutes

Servings: 4 to 6

Happiness has finally arrived!!

Nutrition Information per Serving:

Fats (g): 25.6

Protein (g): 16.3

Net carbs (g): 4.8

Calories: 400

Pinnacle Mug Cake With Berries And Cream

Show time!!

Ingredients:

- 1 Tbsp Swerve
- 1/4 cup of heavy whipping cream
- About 2.5 Tbsp melted ghee
- 2 Tbsp cream cheese
- 1/4 cup of mixed berries
- About 1/2 cup almond flour
- 2 large eggs

Directions:

1. First of all, please make sure you've all the ingredients available. Blend eggs, cream cheese, Swerve, & melted ghee in a blender.
2. Now pour mix into an extra-large, microwave-safe coffee mug.
3. Stir in the berries & almond flour.
4. This step is important. Put the mug inside the cooker, cover, & seal.
5. Use the steam setting, set pressure to high, & cook properly for about 5 to 10 minutes.
6. Then release the steam with quick method, remove the mug, & allow it to cool for about 2 to 5 minutes.

7. One thing remains to be done. Whisk the whipping cream until fluffy.

8. Finally use it to top the cake & serve.

Time to prepare: 10 to 15 minutes

Serves: 4 to 6

Feast for you!!

Nutrition Information per Serving:

15.6g fat

10g protein

13.3g net carbohydrates

Unique Broccoli Soup

Make it quickly.

Ingredients:

- 4 cups chicken stock
- 1 cup coconut cream
- A pinch of salt and white pepper
- 2 cups cheddar cheese (Shredded)
- About 1/2 teaspoon garlic powder
- 1 yellow onion (Chopped)
- 1 cup carrots (Chopped)
- About 2.5 tablespoons ghee (Melted)
- 1 broccoli head, florets separated and roughly chopped

Directions:

1. First of all, please make sure you've all the ingredients available. Now set your instant pot on sauté mode, add ghee, heat it up, add onion, stir and cook properly for about 2 to 5 minutes.
2. One thing remains to be done. Then add carrots, broccoli, stock, garlic powder, salt and pepper, stir, cover and cook properly on High for about 5 to 10 minutes.

3.   Finally add cream and cheese, stir, ladle into bowls & serve.

Preparation time: 10 to 15 minutes

Cooking time: 10 to 15 minutes

Servings: 4 to 7

Supreme level.

Nutrition Information per Serving:

Fat 6

Protein 12

Fiber 7

Carbs 9

Calories 320

Crazy Sausage Shakshuka

A little work here but will be worth it.

Ingredients:

- 4 Eggs
- 1 1/2 cups Water
- 1/3 cup diced Onion
- About 1.5 tbsp Coconut Oil
- 1/2 tsp Salt
- 1/4 tsp Pepper
- 1 tsp Cumin
- About 1.5 tsp Garlic Powder
- 1 Red Bell Pepper (Diced)
- 24 ounces diced Tomatoes
- 3/4 pound Ground Sausage

Directions:

1. Melt the coconut oil in the IP on SAUTE.
2. Add the bell pepper and onion and cook for 3 minutes, until soft.
3. Stir in cumin and garlic powder and cook for another minute.
4. Add the sausage and cook, while breaking it up, for a few minutes.
5. Stir in the tomatoes and transfer the mixture to a greased baking dish.

6. Crack the eggs on top.
7. Next, please pour the water into the Instant Pot and then lower the rack.
8. Place the dish in the IP and close the lid.
9. Cook on HIGH for 10 minutes.
10. Serve and enjoy!

Total Time: 30 to 35 MIN

Serves: 3 to 5

Try it…

Nutrition Information per Serving:

Total Fats 38g

Protein 28g

Net Carbs: 7g

Calories 502

Nostalgic Pesto Scrambled Eggs

Healthy is a new trend these days!! ? Always I guess…

Ingredients:

- About 1.5 tbsp butter or ghee, grass-fed. You can make your own ghee - basil or garlic infused ghee work great! (15g / 0.5 oz)
- Discover foods, kitchen tools and other products i use and love! Find out more
- 1 tbsp pesto (you can make your own green pesto or red pesto) (15g / 0.5 oz)
- Freshly ground black pepper to taste
- About 2.5 tbsp crème fraîche or soured cream or creamed coconut milk (30g / 1.1 oz)
- 3 large eggs, free-range or organic
- Salt to taste (i like pink himalayan salt)

Directions:

1. First of all, please make sure you've all the ingredients available. Crack the eggs into a mixing bowl with a pinch of salt and pepper & beat them well with a whisk or fork.
2. Then pour the eggs into a pan, add butter or ghee & turn the heat on.

3. This step is important. Keep on low heat while stirring constantly.
4. Do not stop stirring as the eggs may get dry & lose the creamy texture. Add the pesto and mix in well.
5. Now take off the heat, spoon crème fraîche in & mix well with the eggs.
6. One thing remains to be done. This will help the eggs cool down & stop cooking while keeping the creamy texture.
7. Finally place on a serving plate & try with sliced avocado on top.

Prep time: 5 to 10 min

Cook time: 5 to 10 min

Total time: 10 to 15 min

Serving: 1 to 2

Stunner!!

Nutrition Information per Serving:

Fat 41.5 grams

Protein 20.4 grams

Net Carbs 2.6 grams

Total Carbs 3.3 grams

Fiber 0.7 grams

Funny Breakfast Omelet

What makes this the best? Check it out for yourself!!

Ingredients:

- 1 teaspoon mustard
- A drizzle of olive oil
- About 1.5 tablespoon homemade mayonnaise
- Salt and black pepper to the taste
- 1 tomato (Chopped)
- 1 small avocado, pitted, peeled and chopped
- About 2.5 bacon slices, cooked and crumbled
- 3 eggs, whisked
- 1 ounces rotisserie chicken (Shredded)

Directions:

1. First of all, please make sure you've all the ingredients available. Then in a bowl, mix eggs with chicken, bacon, mustard, mayo, tomato, avocado, salt and pepper & whisk well.

2. One thing remains to be done. Now set your instant pot on sauté mode, add the oil, heat it up, add eggs mix, spread and cook properly for about 2 to 5 minutes.
3. Finally cover your instant pot, cook your omelet properly on High for about 2 to 5 minutes, divide it between plates & serve for breakfast.

Preparation time: 10 to 15 minutes

Cooking time: 10 to 15 minutes

Servings: 1 to 2

Just got better!!

Nutrition Information per Serving:

Fat 2

Protein 10

Fiber 6

Calories 150

Carbs 8

Iconic Yummiest Glazed Carrot

I bet you'll find it amazing...

Ingredients:

- 2 tablespoons butter
- Dash of hot sauce
- About 2.5 tablespoons Erythritol
- Salt & freshly ground black pepper, to taste
- About 2 tablespoons Dijon mustard
- 1 teaspoon paprika
- About 2.5 teaspoons garlic (Minced)
- 1 teaspoon ground cumin
- 1 pound carrots

Directions:

1. First of all, please make sure you've all the ingredients available. Cut the carrots into quarters lengthwise & then cut each quarter in half.
2. Now arrange the steamer trivet in the bottom of Instant Pot. Add 1 cup of the water in Instant Pot.
3. This step is important. Arrange the carrots on top of trivet.

4. Secure the lid and cook under "Manual" & "High Pressure" for about 2 minutes.

5. Select the "Cancel" and carefully do a Quick release.

6. Then remove the lid & transfer carrots onto a plate.

7. Remove water from Instant Pot.

8. Place the butter in the Instant Pot & select "Sauté". Then add the remaining ingredients & stir to combine.

9. One thing remains to be done. Select the "Cancel" & stir in the carrots.

10. Finally serve warm.

Makes: 4 to 5 servings

Preparation Time: 20 to 30 minutes

Cooking Time: 5 to 10 minutes

The hit list recipe.

Nutritional Information per Serving:

Fat: 6.3g

Protein: 1.6g

Saturated Fat: 3.7g

Sodium: 252mg

Sugar: 13.2g

Carbohydrates: 20.1g

Calories: 108

Dietary Fiber: 3.4g

Fantastic Richly Cheesy Broccoli Soup

Don't forget this one…

Ingredients:

- 2 medium carrots, peeled and chopped
- 1 cup half-and-half
- 1 small yellow onion (Chopped)
- 1/2 cup parmesan cheese (Shredded)
- About 2.5 tablespoons almond flour
- 1 garlic clove (Minced)
- 3 cups homemade vegetable broth
- 1 cup pepper jack cheese (Shredded)
- 5 cups broccoli florets
- About 1.5 teaspoon dill weed
- 1 cup colby jack cheese (Shredded)
- 1 teaspoon smoked paprika
- Salt & freshly ground black pepper, to taste
- 4 American cheese slices, cut into pieces
- 2 tablespoons butter

Directions:

1. First of all, please make sure you've all the ingredients available. Next, please place the butter in the Instant Pot and then select "Sauté".

2. Now add the carrot and onion & cook properly for about 2 to 5 minutes.

3. Stir in flour and garlic & cook properly for about 2 minutes, stirring continuously.

4. This step is important. Stir in broth and cook properly for about 2 minutes or until smooth, stirring continuously.

5. Select the "Cancel" & stir in the broccoli.

6. Then secure the lid & cook under "Manual" and "High Pressure" for about 5 to 10 minutes.

7. Select the "Cancel" and carefully do a Quick release.

8. Now remove the lid & immediately stir in dill weed, paprika, salt and black pepper.

9. One thing remains to be done. Add cheeses and half-and-half & stir until melted and well combined.

10. Finally serve immediately.

Makes: 6 to 7 servings

Preparation Time: 15 to 20 minutes

Cooking Time: 15 to 20 minutes

Amazing cooking starts here...

Nutritional Information per Serving:

Fat: 24.9g

Protein: 17.8g

Saturated Fat: 14g

Sodium: 1018mg

Sugar: 4.2g

Carbohydrates: 13.1g

Calories: 354

Dietary Fiber: 3g

Nostalgic Instant Pot Amazing Beef Stew:

The speed matters...

Ingredients:

- 3 cups of beef broth
- 2 chopped celery ribs
- About 2.5 tablespoons of Worcestershire sauce
- 1 tablespoon of vegetable oil
- 1 diced onion
- 2 bay leaves
- 2 tablespoons of flour
- 1 pound of chopped potatoes
- 3 cloves of minced garlic
- 1 tablespoon of sugar
- About 1.5 tablespoon of salt
- 1 teaspoon of paprika
- 1/2 teaspoon of thyme
- 1/2 teaspoon of thyme
- 1/2 teaspoon of pepper
- About 2 to 3 chopped carrots
- 1 1/2 pounds of lean beef, perfect for stewing. Cut the beef into 1 inch thick chunks for better cooking.
- 1/2 teaspoon of pepper

Directions:

1. First of all, please make sure you've all the ingredients available. Coat the beef chunks with pepper & salt and toss them in flour.
2. Then put oil in Instant Pot and turn the sauté mode.
3. Wait for the oil to be warm enough & then add the beef.
4. Ensure that the beef is brown on all sides. The meat will be a bit caramelized, but take care that the meat does not burn.
5. This step is important. Once one side of the meat is brown & caramelized, turn it for the other side to cook.
6. Pour the beef broth into the pot. Use a wooden spoon to scrape bits from the pit of the pan.
7. Now start adding the Worcestershire sauce, bay leaves, pepper, garlic cloves, salt, thyme, & paprika.
8. Stir well, so that everything is infused properly in the broth.
9. Start adding the other ingredients & continue to stir.

10.   Add the lid of the pot and close the steam valve.

11.   Now you need to press the 'stew/meat' button & set the time to about 35 to 40 minutes in high pressure.

12.   After the stipulated time, let the steam release naturally.

13.   Then after the pressure is released, release the steam valve & wait for a few more minutes before opening the lid.

14.   One thing remains to be done. Add more seasoning if required.

15.   Finally bring out the beef stew & enjoy it with your family and friends!

Serving size: 1.5 cups

Servings per recipe: 4 to 6

Calories: 304 per serving

Calories from fat: 74

Preparation Time: 15 to 20 minutes

Cooking Time: 40 to 45 minutes

Be super

Nutrition Information per Serving:

Saturated fat: 3g

Protein: 30g

Sodium: 845mg

Dietary fiber: 5g

Cholesterol: 72mg

Carbohydrate: 29g

Total fat: 8g

Sugar: 7g

Awesome Cream Cheese Pancakes

Ironic in taste…

Ingredients:

- 1/2 tsp cinnamon
- About 1.5 tbsp butter
- 4 ounces cream cheese
- About 2.5 tsp Swerve
- 4 eggs

Directions:

1. First of all, please make sure you've all the ingredients available. Place everything, except for the butter, in a blender.
2. Then blend until smooth.
3. Melt 1 tsp of the butter in your Instant Pot on sauté.
4. This step is important. Pour half of the pancake batter and cook properly for about 2 to 5 minutes.
5. Now add another teaspoon of batter on top, and flip over.
6. Cook properly for about 2 to 5 minutes more.
7. One thing remains to be done. Repeat with the other pancake.
8. Finally serve & enjoy!

Total Time: 15 to 20 MIN

Serves: 2 to 4

Looking forward to this one!!

Nutrition Information per Serving:

Fat: 34.3 g

Protein: 15.4 g

Net Carbohydrates: 7.4 g

Calories: 376

Great Raspberry Dessert

Simple yet fantastic!!

Ingredients:

- About 3.5 tbsps. stevia
- 1/2 c. coconut oil
- 1/2 c. dried raspberries
- 1/2 c. unsweetened and shredded coconut
- 1/2 c. coconut butter

Directions:

1. First of all, please make sure you've all the ingredients available. Now set your instant pot to sauté mode, add coconut butter, melt it, add coconut, stevia, oil, & raspberries; stir, cover and cook properly on High for about 2 to 5 minutes.
2. Finally spread this on a lined baking sheet, spread well, refrigerate for a couple of hours, slice & serve.

Cooking time: 5 to 10 minutes

Servings: 12 to 14

It is a brand new day…. Ever listened to this one!!

Nutrition Information per Serving:

Protein: 7g

Fats: 5g

Calories: 174

Net carbs: 4g

Perfect Sausage And Peppers

Show time!!

Ingredients:

- 1 15 oz. can tomato sauce
- 2 19 oz. pkg. Italian sausage
- 4 large bell peppers, cut into strips
- 1 c water
- About 1.5 tbsp basil
- 1 tbsp Italian seasoning
- 1 28 oz. can diced tomatoes
- About 2.5 tsp garlic powder

Directions:

1. First of all, please make sure you've all the ingredients available. Place the Italian seasoning, basil, water, garlic powder, tomato sauce, & tomatoes into the Instant Pot.
2. Then put peppers on top. DO NOT MIX.
3. One thing remains to be done. Now close and seal the lid. Set on high for about 25 to 30 minutes. Once done, release the pressure then open the lid.
4. Finally serve & enjoy.

Serves: 5 to 7

Prep: 5 to 10 minutes

Feast for you!!

Nutrition Information per Serving:

Protein: 31g

Net Fat: 43g

Carbohydrates: 10g

Calories: 606

Fantastic Shrimp And Turnips

Light taste.

Ingredients:

- Black pepper
- 1 lb. chopped tomatoes
- 2 lbs. deveined shrimp
- 1 c. water
- Salt
- 3 quartered turnips
- About 4.5 tbsps. olive oil
- Juice of 1 lemon
- 4 chopped onions
- 1 tsp. ground coriander
- 1 tsp. curry powder

Directions:

1. First of all, please make sure you've all the ingredients available. Put the water in your instant pot, add steamer basket, add turnips, cover pot, cook properly on High for about 5 to 10 minutes, drain, transfer to a bowl & leave aside for now.

2. Now clean your instant pot, set it on sauté mode, add oil, heat it up, add onions, stir and cook properly for about 5 to 10 minutes.

3.   This step is important. Add salt, coriander, lemon juice, curry, tomatoes, shrimp and turnips, stir, cover and cook properly on High for about 2 to 5 minutes more.

4.   One thing remains to be done. Then divide shrimp into bowls & serve.

5.   Finally enjoy!

Servings: 4 to 6

Prep time: 10 to 15 minutes

Cook time: 15 to 20 minutes

As the name suggests….

Nutrition Information per Serving:

Fat: 4g

Protein: 15g

Carbs: 7g

Calories: 183

Dashing Kalua Pork

Being super is a matter of recipe… ?

Ingredients:

- 4 lb pork butt
- About 1.5 tbsp liquid smoke
- 1 tbsp olive oil
- 1/2 c water
- About 2.5 tsp salt

Directions:

1. First of all, please make sure you've all the ingredients available. Cut the pork butt in half. Set the cooker on sauté.
2. Then pour the oil & allow to heat. After it's hot, brown the pork.
3. When both halves are browned, turn the pot off & add liquid smoke and water.
4. This step is important. Place roasts into the pot then sprinkle with salt.
5. Now close and seal the lid. Set on high for about 85 to 90 minutes.
6. When timer sounds, naturally release the pressure for about 20 to 25 minutes. Remove the lid.
7. Take the meat out & shred. Throw away any fat.

8. One thing remains to be done. Then add juices to the pot to keep the meat moist.
9. Finally serve over riced cauliflower.

Serves: 10 to 12

Prep: 5 to 10 minutes

Being a legend.

Nutrition Information per Serving:

Protein: 36g

Net Fat: 30g

Carbohydrates: 0g

Calories: 415

Delightful Beef Meatloaf

Magical…

Ingredients:

- 1/4 c. grated parmesan
- 1/2 c. beef stock
- 1/4 c. chopped yellow onion
- 1 whisked egg
- 1 c. keto ketchup
- Salt
- Black pepper
- About 1.5 chopped yellow onion
- 1 tbsp. minced garlic
- 1/2 tsp. dried thyme
- About 1.5 tbsp. olive oil
- 2 lbs. ground beef

Directions:

1. First of all, please make sure you've all the ingredients available. In a bowl, mix beef with cheese, 1/4 cup onion, egg, thyme, salt and pepper & stir really well.
2. Then set your instant pot on sauté mode, add the oil, heat it up, and 1 yellow onion, stir and cook properly for about 2 to 5 minutes.

3.   This step is important. Add stock and ketchup, stir and cook properly for about 2 minutes more.
4.   Now shape a round meatloaf out of the beef mix, add it to the pot, cover and cook properly on High for about 15 to 20 minutes.
5.   One thing remains to be done. Divide meatloaf on plates, drizzle the sauce from the pot all over & serve.
6.   Finally enjoy!

Servings: 4 to 5

Prep time: 10 to 15 minutes

Cooking time: 20 to 30 minutes

Right on track.

Nutrition Information per Serving:

Fat: 6g

Protein: 14g

Carbs: 8g

Calories: 363

Reliable Ribs With Coleslaw

When you're fantastic, this is best!!

Ingredients:

Ribs:

- 1/2 tsp dry mustard
- About 1 tsp salt
- 2.5 lbs. baby back ribs
- 3/4 tsp black pepper
- 1 c favorite barbecue sauce
- 1 tsp onion powder
- 1/2 tsp garlic powder
- About 1 tsp chili powder
- 1/2 tsp paprika

Coleslaw:

- 1/4 c apple cider vinegar
- Salt
- 1/2 head red cabbage
- Pepper
- About 2.5 shredded carrots
- 2 tbsp sweetener of choice
- 1 c mayonnaise
- 1 small head cabbage

Directions:

1. First of all, please make sure you've all the ingredients available. Make the rub for ribs: Mix chili powder, dry mustard, pepper, paprika, garlic powder, salt, and onion powder.
2. Now stir to combine.
3. Cut the ribs into pieces, so they will fit in the Instant Pot.
4. This step is important. Stacking is okay. Coat ribs with dry rub.
5. Next, quickly add one inch of water to the bottom. Also please place a trivet inside. Stack ribs on the trivet. Close & seal the lid. Set on high for about 15 to 20 minutes.
6. Then while the ribs are cooking make the coleslaw: Put cabbage and carrots in large bowl. In a smaller bowl, mix the pepper, sweetener, salt, apple cider vinegar, and mayonnaise.
7. Stir well to combine. Pour over cabbage & stir well to coat.
8. Refrigerate until serving.
9. When the ribs are done, quick release the pressure.
10. Then put ribs on a plate. Remove the trivet & discard the liquid.
11. Add some barbecue sauce to the bottom of the pot & add some ribs, more

sauce, more ribs, repeat until all the ribs and the sauce have been used.

12.   Now close and seal the lid. Set on high & cook properly for about 10 to 15 minutes.

13.   One thing remains to be done. Quick release the pressure & put ribs on the serving plates.

14.   Finally serve with coleslaw and enjoy.

Serves: 4 to 6

Prep: 30 to 35 minutes

Being rich is a plus point ?

Nutrition Information per Serving:

Protein: 37g

Net Fat: 76g

Carbohydrates: 19g

Calories: 958

Super Easy Pork Roast

Believe me…

Ingredients:

- About 1.5 tbsp. olive oil
- 4 lbs. pork shoulder
- 1/4 c. keto Jamaican spice mix
- 1/2 c. beef stock

Directions:

1. First of all, please make sure you've all the ingredients available. In a bowl, mix pork with oil & spice mix and rub well.
2. Then set your instant pot on sauté mode, add pork & brown for a few minutes on each side.
3. Add stock, cover pot & cook pork shoulder on High for about 40 to 45 minutes.
4. One thing remains to be done. Now slice roast & serve.
5. Finally enjoy!

Servings: 12 to 14

Prep time: 10 to 15 minutes

Cook time: 45 to 50 minutes

Always kept wondering how it was made... One day I sat beside my chef and got it.

Nutrition Information per Serving:

Fat: 6g

Protein: 16g

Carbs: 10g

Calories: 400

Charming Chicken Chili Verde

Amazing cooking starts here…

Ingredients:

- About 1.5 tbsp whole cumin seed
- 3 lb. bone-in skinless chicken thighs
- 1 medium onion
- 1 tbsp fish sauce
- 4 tomatillos, husks removed (Quartered)
- 2 Serrano chilies, stem removed, rough chopped
- 2 poblano peppers, seeds and stem removed, rough chopped
- 1/2 c cilantro leaves
- 2 Anaheim peppers, seeds and stem removed, rough chopped
- About 6.5 cloves garlic, peeled
- Salt

Directions:

1. First of all, please make sure you've all the ingredients available. Place cumin, garlic, tomatillos, onion, peppers, and chicken in the Instant Pot.
2. Now sprinkle generously with salt.
3. Heat on high until simmering. Close and seal the lid.

4. This step is important. Set on high and cook properly for about 10 to 15 minutes. Quick release the pressure.
5. Carefully remove the chicken & place on a plate.
6. Then add fish sauce and cilantro.
7. Blend with immersion blender until as smooth as you like it.
8. Taste & adjust seasoning if needed.
9. Then put the chicken back in the cause.
10. One thing remains to be done. You can shred chicken if you would like or leave pieces whole.
11. Finally place in a bowl & add cilantro and lime wedge. Serve and enjoy.

Serves: 5 to 6

Prep: 10 to 15 minutes

Don't forget this one…

Nutrition Information per Serving:

Protein: 45g

Net Fat: 9g

Carbohydrates: 8g

Calories: 297

Thanks for reading my book.